The 8 Secrets That Will Destroy The
copyright 2016 Dr.Christa .

MW00955324

Dr.Christa Krzeminski
1800 W. Hillsboro Blvd.
Ste. 212
Deerfield Beach, Fl 33442
(954) 570-5848

DrChrista@DrChrista.com

You should not construe the information in this book as a substitute or replacement for medical advice for your specific health issues. This book is designed to provide competent and reliable information regarding the subject matters covered. However, it is sold with the understanding that the author is not engaged in rendering specific health recommendations and diagnoses or other medical advice. Laws and practices often vary from state to state and if other health attention is required, the services of a health care provider should be sought. The author disclaims any liability that is incurred from the use and/or application of the contents of this book.

Enjoy!
John & Christie DiLemme

* This is one of our clients books. Thought you would like it!

Table of Contents

Introduction

Diet is the most powerful influence over your health. Making basic changes and transitioning to a plant based lifestyle you can certainly expect great health changes. The information in this book is not meant to diagnose or treat a particular illness. Rather, the intention is to expose you to the absolute potential you have on a daily basis to provide your body with the most powerful medicine in existence- the proper food. Your body is the ultimate healing machine. It is up to you on what level you want to function.

This book serves as important food for thought! What you consume will have the most inspiring or the most devastating impact on your health. Every morsel of food consumed has a result. This book is meant to stir you up and give you the motivation to seek out the best food choices possible. I do not put people on medications and I certainly do not recommend taking them off. I am not telling you what to do, rather I am exposing you to information you need to make healthy choices. The information in this book is purposed to further the health dialogue between you and your health professionals; it is certainly not meant to be a substitute.

Eating healthy is simple and delicious. It is the one aspect of your health that you completely control. Enjoy this book and absolutely love your health transformation!

About The Author

Dr.Christa's passion and thirst for nutrition knowledge started during her high school years when she was always searching for the right combination of foods to eat before a track meet or soccer game. These curiosities lead Dr.Christa to earn a Bachleor of Science in Chemistry from the State University of New York at Oneonta. It was during her undergraduate studies she began studying the pioneers of the biochemistry and nutrition world- Dr.C Colin Campbell, Nathan Pritikin, Dr. Caldwell Esselstyn and Dr. Dean Ornish.

The evidence was there, the literature was packed with how food and nutrition changes health! The road to change people's lives was just beginning. Dr.Christa earned her doctorate of chiropractic medicine from New York Chiropractic College as well as a fellowship in acupuncture. Dr.Christa owns and operates a nutrition and holistic medicine center in south Florida. She instills in patients the foundation of health is and always be what you eat. She designs personalized food and nutrition plans that are absolutely simplified for each of her patients. She has successfully changed the lives and health of many kids, moms, weekend warriors and elite and professional athletes. Dr.Christa believes that your health care providers should lead you on the path of health which is free of disease, medication and full of life, vibrancy and longevity.

To speak with Dr.Christa directly or to book her for a speaking engagement or an interview, please call (954) 570-5848 or email DrChrista@DrChrista.com

Chapter 1:   Just because You Are Skinny Does Not Mean You Are Healthy

One of the deadliest flaws in society's view of health is, *skinny people are always healthy*. So, this flawed logic leads people to think "well, if I just lose 40 pounds, if I were just thin, all of my health issues will miraculously disappear!" Even many doctors, at the first sign of high blood pressure, cholesterol issues, migraines or my personal favorite, "pre-diabetes", tell their patients just lose weight and the conversation stops there! Does a number on a scale or a dress size really indicate health? Will jumping on the next fad diet really make your "pre-diabetes" go away? Has a skinny person ever had a heart attack, thyroid issue or cancer?

Being skinny does not guarantee health.
Appearances can be very deceiving. Plastic surgery, fad diets, rounds of chemotherapy and radiation are all roads that lead to "skinny". Do any of them result in optimal health and longevity? Plastic surgery and fad diets are all quick fixes. They are temporary solutions for those who are impatient, lazy and unrealistic. This is an incredibly deadly false sense of security.

Health is not just the absence of disease. Health also includes not taking any medications, feeling great, looking younger than ever, and having more energy, less pain and better sleep. Your health is a direct result of the food you put in your mouth. **It truly is that simple**. Do you want better health AND a smaller waistline? It is all in the food you eat over the long term- no short term solutions here!! Let's take a look at the 4 biggest "skinny fads." Listening to them can destroy your health.

***You're So Skinny, You Can Eat Whatever You
Want*.......** Wow- this is so wrong and yet how many times
have you heard this said, perhaps about you, or have you
said it about someone you know. NO ONE can eat
whatever they want. No one can eat junk food, go to the
drive thru, live on cheesecake, wine, beer, hamburgers,
chicken wings and steak and honestly have the expectation
of good health. This is one of those times in life when it
sounds too good to be true and it actually is.

Everyone is built in their own unique way. We all have
our own blueprint. People are all shapes and sizes.
Securing good health is not just about a number on a
scale. Many people are very thin on the outside and have a
huge mess going on inside! It should not be shocking when
people who live on processed food, junk food, take out and
the drive thru end up always sick. Your co-worker who is
skinny as a rail and always sick, coughing, taking a new
prescription and missing work to go to the doctor is not the
person you should aspire to be.

Would you be utterly astonished when your car ran out
of gas and just completely stopped running, because there
was not even a drop of gas in the gas tank? Of course this
is not shocking. You have no reasonable expectation or
right to expect health when you choose to run on empty.
Would you be shocked if you put diesel fuel in a car that
required unleaded and the car wouldn't even run**? Do any
of these car examples have anything to do with what
the car looks like on the outside**? You can own the top
of the line, pinnacle of luxury, Bentley and should you
decide to not put oil in the engine, and put soda in the gas
tank instead of high octane gasoline your result would be a

ruined engine and a car that won't move out of the garage. The results would not be shocking. Sadly, no one would ever treat a car like that.

Yet, the majority of Americans are on 4+ medications, sick, tired and standing idle while their health deteriorates. That security blanket of "I am skinny" means very little. Fuel, nutrients, the essence of great health and a prosperous life lies in the food you consume. It is rather simple, high octane fuel in means high performance output. Be very careful when you ask someone who is "skinny" for health advice. If you hear the words "I can eat anything and never gain a pound", you could very well be receiving very dangerous, health destroying advice.

Keep It Under 1200 Calories... Counting calories is the biggest weight loss fad in the diet industry. Unfortunately, it is usually the only advice many doctors give to patients when they are dealing with high blood pressure, type II diabetes, thyroid issues and obesity. Calorie restrictions or more accurately, starvation plans, are incredibly dangerous.

If losing weight was just a matter of restricting calories for a week or two, we would be a society of fit, trim and healthy people. Take a look around, society is far from that! Health and weight control are not related to the quantity of calories consumed, rather there is a direct correlation to the quality of calories consumed. You can consume 1200 calories per day of drive thru, processed food that is loaded with fat, sodium, hydrogenated oils, sugar and other artificial sweeteners and dyes and you would still stay fat and sick.

You can consume 2500 calories of whole food plant based starch loaded foods and be medication free, disease free, fit and trim. One of the most significant issues that result from decades of crash dieting and calorie restriction is thyroid dysfunction. Depriving the body of needed energy and nutrients will essentially "burn out" the thyroid.

Carbs Make You Fat... Thanks to fad diets like the Atkins Diet, the deadly and disease promoting high protein diets have taken root. Every fitness center in America pays homage to the high protein diet. This notion that carbs are bad and make you gain weight is absolutely 1000% false and NOT supported by ANY professional research.

Our metabolism is designed to use glucose as its main energy and readily store chains of glucose in the liver and throughout the musculoskeletal system for quick energy on demand. It is a brilliant design. High protein diets work by making you sick. They starve the body of its preferred energy source, which is carbohydrates, and force the system into a state of ketosis.

Ketosis is an emergency metabolic process which the body obtains its energy from ketone bodies as opposed to glucose or through glycolysis. Simply stated, the body will get its energy from fats or protein. Ketosis is a state of sickness for the body. It is a backup plan. This plan kicks in when the emergency light goes off. Our metabolism was not built to run on ketone bodies. **Running this back up metabolism comes at a very steep cost to your health**.

Initially, you will experience a TEMPORARY weight loss. You will also experience an enormous strain on the liver and heart. The LONG TERM result of sustained ketosis is serious. High blood pressure, very high cholesterol, kidney stones, kidney failure, liver failure, type II diabetes, irritable bowel syndrome, severe body odor, bad breath, dehydration, cancer and weakened heart muscle are just a **few of the guarantees afforded by long term high protein food plans**.

The research is clear and has been for decades. High protein diets cause disease. Plant based foods provide us with carbohydrates. Not only do these foods such as fruits, vegetables, lentils, seeds, nuts and beans, give us energy, they also provide many life sustaining nutrients. Fiber, vitamins, minerals and antioxidants are naturally found in plant based foods. The starches such as potatoes, sweet potatoes, squash, rice, corn, quinoa, are especially crucial in building long term health.

As an added bonus for many, they CERTAINLY do allow for excellent weight control. *So, absolutely, positively YES you can lose weight while eating a whole food plant based starch dominated food plan, the research PROVES it!*

Who Needs Food- Just Give Me An Energy Drink..
Energy drinks are deadly. People have literally had fatal heart attacks from drinking 5-6 energy drinks and then working out. Unfortunately, energy drinks are also the favorite appetite suppressant for many desperate people. In a delusional effort to stay "skinny" so many people, especially young women, consume energy drinks in place of meals.

Energy drinks are nothing but a crazy mixture of stimulants. They have no nutritional value. They are not healthy. Most importantly, they can be very dangerous. A stimulant will excite the nervous system. It will increase heart rate and the rate of breathing, raise blood pressure and effect kidney function.

The label, energy drink, is completely misleading. These cocktails do not provide the body with energy. They absolutely do not nourish the body. **The sole source of energy for the body is healthy food.** Want energy for a workout? Eat a banana or orange. Falling short of energy in the afternoon? Boost the nutritional value of your lunch and snacks – add more plant based foods and starch!

Artificial sweeteners and caffeine do not provide energy- they provide a heart attack. They artificially stimulate the body much like drugs do. Use of energy drinks to lose weight is one of the most recent fads. Many young women, even teenagers resort to energy drinks as a form of quick weight loss. Unfortunately, the cost of quick weight loss may be a lifelong heart or kidney issue.

YOUR health is the result of YOUR daily consistent food choices. Want to get rid of your blood pressure meds, lose weight, gain more energy, sleep better and look amazing? Change the food you are eating! Health is not a number on a scale or the size of your pants; it is the internal disease fighting power developed from the food you eat!

Chapter 2- Stop Prostate Cancer, Breast Cancer, High Cholesterol, Acne, Irritable Bowel Syndrome By Getting Rid Of This....

What is so bad for you that it should be considered public health enemy #1? *The answer unequivocally is dairy*. Our society was raised to believe dairy is healthy; it is needed to build strong bones. Nothing could be further from the truth.

Dairy is the root of many diseases. Decades of research points to the destructiveness of the fat, protein, foreign growth factors and the foreign white blood cells in dairy products. Yet, we believe all of the"got milk" commercials. Eliminating dairy from your food plan will ultimately save your life. The research and proof is there and has been since the 1940's.

The dairy industry has done a brilliant job of hiding the truth, side stepping the research and promoting cancer causing foods as vital for life! The dairy industry is not intentionally trying to harm us, it is just business. People do not stop and consider the dangers of dairy simply because they were never told about them. Below are the 5 deadly dairy fallacies that the dairy industry does not want you to know....

1.)Dairy is a good source of calcium.... Calcium is a vital nutrient. It is needed to add strength to bones and teeth, help muscles contract and relax, balance fluids in and outside of cells, sending and receiving nerve signals, releasing many hormones and keeping the heart beating normally. We cannot survive without this wonderful mineral. It makes perfect sense to make sure your foods contain adequate forms of calcium. "Drink milk- it builds strong bones"- has long been the anthem for the dairy industry. After all, milk contains about 300 mg of calcium per cup. It seems logical that adding dairy to your food plan will provide you with that all important crucial mineral, calcium.

Unfortunately, this is totally false. You are saying, "how could that be?" "The body needs calcium, milk has lots of it, why would my body not benefit from milk?" Not only will your body not benefit from the calcium, as we will see in a moment, your body could suffer disease from long term use of dairy. First, let's take a look at dairy.

Long touted, the savior of bones, because of its high calcium content, dairy DOES NOT help bones. As a matter of fact, its high acid load allows for a tremendous loss of calcium thru the kidneys.(1) Think about this for one moment, the high amount of calcium in dairy is precisely what a developing calf needs to grow. After all, that is why nature constructed dairy the way it did- to accommodate the needs of growth and development for cows. Cow milk is for cows!!!

If high doses of calcium built strong bones we would have to believe that the huge mega blocks of calcium made its way through your gut wall with ease. Much in the way water flows thru a colander. Basic physiology and anatomy teaches us differently. The gut is not a passive membrane. It is actually very selective. This is for our own good.

Could you imagine if calcium and other minerals and toxins freely flowed thru the gut to the rest of the body?

Your soft tissue would harden or calcify and your body would become polluted and toxic. The gut is designed to allow only small amounts of calcium thru to the rest of the body.

So, understanding the gut is selective and that high amounts of calcium could actually cause blood vessels and other tissues to harden, why would we believe that drinking a cup of calcium loaded milk would build strong bones? So, mega dosing on calcium is never the answer to building strong anything in the body. The idea that drinking milk and eating yogurt and cheese is healthy and is necessary for growth, development and ultimately the maintenance of bones is a **seriously flawed idea** and at its root does not make any sense. It has created great commercials for the dairy industry.

Many pediatricians still believe children need milk for growth and development. This seems like it goes against nature. There is no debating that human babies absolutely 1000% need human breast milk to grow and thrive. It is why mothers produce breast milk, to feed and nourish their young. Human breast milk is loaded with antibodies to protect a new born and it is PERFECTLY formulated with the right vitamins, minerals and nutrients for a new born. Nobody will debate the importance of breast feeding.

Current medical research and literature supports breast feeding infants for at least 3 months. Many professionals and new moms believe that breast feeding for 6-12 months is ideal. I am not debating the length of time infants should be breastfed, I am making the point that it is certainly unanimous, breast feeding is the best choice for providing a newborn with all of the antibodies, vitamins, minerals and nutrients needed to get off to a healthy start. We all agree that moms do not need to do anything special to produce the incredibly nourishing breast milk. The human body is amazing in its innate ability to know exactly how to produce breast milk.

Now, if breast milk is perfect for human newborns, it should comes as no surprise that cow's milk-dairy- is uniquely produced for cows! It has the right amount of vitamins, minerals and nutrients for cows. The amount of calcium in cow's milk is exactly what a calf needs. The amount of calcium in breast milk is exactly what a human needs to support growth and development.

In case you are wondering what the difference in calcium content is, I will tell you. Cow's milk contains 300 mg per cup and human breast milk contains 80 mg per cup. So, at the point in life when the human body grows and develops at its highest rate, the amount of calcium required for humans is a fraction of what is required by cows! What does this have to do with dairy? This high calcium wonder drink is not going to deliver any health saving calcium. Our bodies do not require nor can they use the high levels of calcium in dairy, **we are not cows, so why do we expect to benefit from their milk?**

Where Do Cow's Get Their Calcium?

Have you ever wondered why dairy is a good source of calcium? How did cows get so lucky to have so much calcium in their milk? Many people believe cows make calcium. This is absolutely not the case. Calcium is neither created nor destroyed in the cow's body, and in our bodies too. Calcium is a wonderful mineral created by the earth. It is found in soil. Cows obtain their calcium supply from the grass they eat.

So, if an enormous animal such as a cow can get more than enough calcium from grass, why do we need to consume large quantities of dairy to get our calcium? I strongly suggest and encourage you to go right for the plants! Plants absorb calcium along with other minerals from the soil through their root systems. As the plant grows and matures, these minerals are incorporated into the plant. Choose a plant based diet.

The calcium available in plants is very easily utilized by our bodies. It allows for more than enough calcium to maintain great health. The push by the dairy industry to sell the idea that milk is great for strong bones is a marketing effort. The dairy industry through its Dairy Management Incorporated, spent $210.7 MILLION dollars in 2013 to fund its own biased research and market dairy to consumers.(2) This is an incredibly powerful industry who is focused on one goal and one goal only- PROFITS.

The dairy industry in no way, shape or form is concerned about health and longevity. All of the current research on calcium and bone health is funded by the dairy industry. Many prominent physicians researchers, like Dr.T.Colin Campbell and Dr. John A. McDougall, have cautioned the general public on research that is so heavily biased. So, if you drink milk or eat yogurt and cheese for the calcium, you should stop immediately! It is not working!

Here's one final note on calcium. Again, we are back to the calcium in cow's milk that is designed for cows-humans do not possess the enzymes and other intrinsic factors needed to properly utilize calcium in dairy. ***We do however, metabolize and utilize the calcium found in spinach, chia seeds, quinoa and oranges very easily!*** Calcium is readily available in most plant based foods. If cows can get their calcium from plants than so can humans!

2.) Total Acid Overload... The idea that acid is bad for the body and leads to disease has come into vogue in recent years. Everybody is talking about high acid and the need to reduce acid in the diet. Many people understand that high acid is bad, they just do not know what foods constitute high acid foods.

Much of this is the result of cancer research pointing to the fact that cancer cells seem to love an acidic environment and cannot proliferate at all in a more alkaline environment. This is tremendous news! Many diseases we see today have their root in an acidic environment. Consider this, GERD, acid reflux, gastritis (most affectionately called "sour stomach"), gall stones, kidney stones, osteoporosis and of course, cancer all live at 1000 Acid Drive. In other words, they cannot exist if the environment in the body is not acidic.

You are more than likely wondering "what does this have to do with my milk, yogurt, cheese and ice cream?" Well, it is not too tough to understand that the more acidic foods you eat, the more acidic your body's internal environment/chemistry will be. Conversely, the more alkaline or basic your food is the more alkaline or basic your body will be.

So, let me just hit this one out of the park right off the bat, cheese is the most acidic food the western diets boasts and it is consumed in monstrous portions! **I want to make one extremely important point here,** dairy is high in protein and protein is made up of chains of amino acids. Amino acids are acidic- very acidic! Dairy is a very acidic food.

I often will laugh when I hear a patient tell me his/her gastroenterologist recommended decreasing the acidic foods such as tomatoes, lemons and peppers to help combat GERD. Never a mention of meat, cheese or dairy!!!! This high acid load is very destructive. Consuming high acid foods over an extended period of time is a slow steady acidic assault. This is the foundation for massive disease over a lifetime.

It is all preventable by just simply not consuming dairy. When your doctor tells you to reduce the acidic foods in your diet, the first food that needs to be eliminated is dairy.

3.)Why is milk white? Have you ever wondered why milk is so creamy white? We all have seen the "Got Milk" commercials with athletes sporting the white milk mustache. For moms that have nursed their young, you know breast milk is not that brilliant pearly white. So, why is milk, yogurt and cheese white?

Many in the food and dairy industry will have you believe it is from the high calcium content (that we all now know is dangerous). To some degree, this is true. The calcium will give it somewhat of a white color. Get ready, I am going to raise the gross factor by quite a bit here. The white color of dairy comes from the high amount of white blood cells in the product! Let's visit breast milk one more time. Human breast milk is tremendous in passing along immunity to a new born. Well, cow's milk has the same intention for its young. Passing along immunity is vital for a young calf and one form that immunity is white blood cells.

Unfortunately, these white blood cells are downright harmful for humans. The numbers of antibodies in milk is quite startling. The "acceptable" level of white blood cells in milk is 750,000 per cc of milk. Keep in mind, that one cc is 1/3 of an ounce! It should alarm you that there is actually an acceptable level, now, if you can forgive that, let's see just how many white blood cells from a cow are being mixed into your cereal in the morning or are in that slice of cheese on your turkey sandwich for lunch.

With 750,000 antibodies per 1/3 of an ounce, the average slice of cheese is 2 ounces that is 4,500,000 white blood cells in that single slice of cheese!! In your morning cereal, the average amount of milk used is 1 cup which is 8 ounces. That is 18,000,000 white blood cells in your morning cereal! As, humans, we cannot use the white blood cells to fight our diseases. As a matter of fact, our body-our own immune system, recognizes these white blood cells as foreign invaders and fights to eliminate them. Mixing antibodies and immune factors from dairy with our own is a **recipe for auto immune issues** and an immune system that could certainly face unique challenges and weaken.

Also adding to the brilliant white of milk are many hormones that are natural to the cow. Growth hormones, insulin and insulin growth factors are found in milk. These hormones once consumed *cause an increase in our own hormonal activity.* One particularly dangerous hormone that is passed on through the consumption of dairy is insulin like growth factor 1.

IGF1 is a hormone that our bodies produce as needed. IGF1 is responsible for causing growth of tissue and cells. The increase in consumption of milk and the increase in consumption of animal protein will cause an increase in IGF1 in our bodies. This has been directly correlated to the formation and progression of lung, breast, prostate and colon cancers (3).

4.) Linked to cardiovascular disease, prostate cancer and juvenile diabetes. Dairy is high in fat and cholesterol, especially saturated fat. Cheese is the most notable offender. Many realize the dangers of red meat and have wisely eliminated red meat from their food plan. It is wonderful that many people now make the connection between red meat and poor health. It seems folks find it an easy transition in limiting and ultimately eliminating red meat from their food plans.

They marvel at watching their cholesterol, blood pressure and weight drop. It is easy to see- literally you can see how much fat is in cuts of steak. So, logically, if you eat less stuff with fat then you may actually improve health. This is absolutely true- if you eat less fat you will wear less fat. This is the favorite advice of many cardiologists- get your cholesterol and weight down- skip the steak and you should be fine.

Getting rid of red meat from your food plan is a great place to start your weight control journey- yes, it is a starting point. To continue on the journey of health, we must also identify other food factors that need to be changed. The next logical food to eliminate is dairy.

Remember, it is easy to see how red meat is a villain. **Well, folks dairy is essential liquid meat!** Same animal, same nutrients, same poor health results! It really is not a stretch to understand. Cholesterol is found exclusively in animal products, this includes dairy. So, consuming more animal products will lead to more cholesterol in the blood. To lower cholesterol, simply limit animal products. Dairy is an animal product.

There is no need to worry about not getting enough cholesterol. The body can make its own, it is essential to many functions in the body. With this in mind, the body does what it does best- protect itself, heal and get healthier. Making cholesterol is one of the jobs of the liver. Cholesterol is a substance needed to protect our organs and make hormones and other substances needed to be healthy. What the body needs, the body can make.

One function the body is not very efficient in performing is the elimination of excess cholesterol. So, when we add a lot of extra cholesterol through the consumption of dairy and other animal products, the excess is stored in our blood vessels, around our organs and underneath the skin. This excess cholesterol is dangerous and facilitates many disease processes, including cancer. (4)

5.) What is the big deal about antibiotic and hormone free- You cannot make it out of the dairy section in the grocery store without seeing this overabundance of advertising for "Hormone and antibiotic free- no added hormones"- you say to yourself, "well that must be a good thing- it makes sense, the less garbage added to my food, the better it must be" That is absolutely correct- the less added stuff the better. This advertisement is placed on many dairy, meat and poultry products. *Unfortunately, when it comes to dairy, the danger does not lie in what is added, it lies in what is naturally found in the milk.*

Milk is naturally nasty and in its natural state is harmful to human health. Don't blame nature, remember, cow's milk was created to nourish cows not humans. We spoke about the natural antibodies found in milk. What is also found in milk and all dairy products are the hormones natural to the cow. Those hormones are needed by the animal for its own needs.

Think about it, animals need and produce their own hormones and it would seem likely to find those hormones in the products that are consumed. As for dairy specifically, the most dangerous hormone NATURALLY produced by cows and found in cow's milk is insulin like growth factor I or IGF1. IGF1 is responsible for increasing the rate of growth. As is expected, it is found in cow's milk in the appropriate amount for a growing calf.

A calf will grow from 50 pounds to more than 600 pounds in 6-7 months. Humans on the other hand will grow from 7 pounds to, on average, 170 pounds in 18 years. You can clearly see, the rate of growth for a calf is much different than that of a human.

The rapid growth of cows would require growth factors that humans do not. One such growth factor is IGF1. There is no way to produce milk without hormones. They are naturally there! So what is with all of this advertising of no added hormones? Well, it is common practice in the dairy and meat industry to give cows additional hormones- steroids- to grow faster and produce more milk. This practice is strictly profit based.

There are definitely products on the market that have added growth hormones and other steroids that were given to the animal and found their way into the milk. *Research has clearly shown the hormones in milk products certainly contribute to inflammation, prostate issues, hormonal or breast issues and gastrointestinal issues*.(**5**) How is it that we are lead to believe that it is the added hormones (which are actually the same hormones found naturally in milk!!) that are the source of the illness and not the IGF1 found in even organic milk? Once again, an industry is banking on the general public being too dumb to ask that question!

How would you like to live on bean burritos, veggie pizza, pasta and bagels?

Now for some absolutely fantastic news- this high protein low carb fad is a complete lie. There is not one legitimate, unbiased research study that supports long term high protein eating is a healthy eating plan which provides superior health and longevity. As you have seen, the research clearly demonstrates the opposite. Eating is fun, yummy and of course, the foundation of health. **There is no such thing as deprivation on a whole food plant based starch dominated food plan.** Mashed potatoes, corn, veggie pizza, pasta with delicious marinara sauce, banana ice cream and apple pie are just a few of the typical foods consumed on plant powered food plans! It is really quite simple to get started.

First, allow me to give you a few quick and easy substitutions. Replace your skim, 2% and whole milk with almond, cashew or rice milk. Most grocery stores carry these substitutes and in many instances you will find almond and cashew milk in the dairy section! Next, stop with the yogurt, yes, and even Greek yogurt. There are non dairy based yogurts that taste great. They are made from coconut milk or soy milk. Now, for the ice cream. There are coconut based frozen desserts available that taste better than ice cream.

Take it up a notch; I have included my favorite banana ice cream recipe in the recipe section of the book! Sprouted bagels with nut butter, veggie pizza with NO CHEESE, rice and bean burritos, vegetable soup, sweet potatoes and hummus are just a few incredible foods that you should be eating daily!

Chapter 3: Everyone is a protein Expert....The Most Deadly Advice You Are Receiving...

Protein, protein, protein- where do you get your protein? I am asked this absolutely insane question at least 100 times per week! The worry and concern over protein is mind boggling. People are so focused on protein that they have no true understanding of what they are actually saying!

The conditioned concern is where are you getting your animal tissue from! Everyone is an expert- you need lean protein to build strong bones and muscles and to stay healthy. Well, facts don't lie and we are absolutely a nation of sick and obese people. It is time for a health revolution. It is time to start building health, curing disease and living long, healthy and prosperous lives. **The core of this is not nor will it ever be animal protein**.

Have you ever heard or read of a case of death by protein deficiency? I can assure you, in this great country there is not one case of dietary protein deficiency. However, there are a myriad of individuals who fall victim to health issues **that are the result of overconsumption of protein.**

Take a trip to Japan, China or any other Asian country and you will find people are lean, healthy and fit. Obesity, cancer, high blood pressure, kidney disease, lupus, multiple sclerosis and osteoporosis are not part of their everyday lives. When you look closer you will definitely see the truth, their diets are based on starch- rice! No dominance of animal products!!

Whole food plant based food plans with starch as the dominating force is the recipe to build health and completely annihilate disease. This article will expose the danger of protein....keep reading, you will discover the shocking truth about protein and it will save your life!

Just The Basics...

There are 3 vital nutrients that all living things- plants or animals- need to create and sustain life. Those irreplaceable nutrients are the macronutrients, proteins, fats and carbohydrates. We need ALL of them! While protein is a bit of the supreme ruler, all of the macronutrients are needed for growing and for overall health. They have very unique responsibilities in the body and great health cannot be achieved if we do not have these nutrients in the correct amounts.

The right balance is the key. So often, we believe health and disease are related to some sort of deficiency- iron deficiency, vitamin D deficiency, essential fatty acid deficiency- the key is what leads to the deficiency, why is there a deficiency? Were we short changed on a nutrient or was it a situation of gross overages of something creating a toxic situation?

So many illness and diseases we suffer from have a root in an overconsumption of protein. This theme of high protein low carb eating is devastating. It literally sets the table for diseases such as heart disease, cancer, thyroid issues, irritable bowel syndrome, hormonal imbalance, osteoporosis and many others. Let's take a look at the truth about protein.

We Can't Live Without It.... Protein is vital for life.
Protein has many different jobs in the human body. First, proteins are the work horse of the cells. Their jobs vary from cell to cell. Proteins help in maintaining the structure of cells, they transport different substances from one cell to another, they act as a storage container for amino acids and they are important components of enzymes and hormones. But wait, it gets better! Proteins also help make up the part of muscles that contract, they are crucial parts of antibodies, they replicate DNA, in short, proteins participate in every aspect of every cell in the body!(6)

So this begs the questions, what is a protein? A protein is defined as a class of nitrogenous organic compounds that consist of large molecules composed of one or more long chain amino acids and are an essential part of all living organisms. There are 20 amino acids we need to build protein and 9 of them are essential, meaning that the human body cannot produce them so they must be provided through food.

The 11 non essential amino acids can be produced in the body (7). So, getting the essential amino acids through food is very important. This is a big concept to understand. Protein is critical, the issue becomes how much and what food sources are the best? This is where it all starts to break down and it has over the last few centuries.

For many, protein is synonymous with meat. This word association is deadly. It is true, most meat is certainly high in protein, the two words are hardly interchangeable. This misconception has been handed down through the centuries.

Protein was first discovered in 1839. Soon after, early scientists such as Carl Voit and Max Rubner, became advocates of high protein. This was not because of any research proving that humans needed mega amounts of protein. Quite the contrary, Voit actually found, through research, that man needs 48.5 grams of protein per day! Keep in mind one meal of lentils, rice and beans provide 32-37 grams of protein! However, he went on to recommend 118 grams per day. (8)

Why the huge discrepancy? The answer is it was purely cultural- meat , which was equated to protein, was a status symbol. This cultural bias became entrenched in society. If you were wealthy and cultured you ate meat. If you were simple, uneducated, lazy and poor you ate foods like potatoes and corn. This arrogance dominated much of the research and opinions of society for many years. This, unfortunately, was also the basis for many early governmental recommendations regarding protein.

Even today meat is somewhat of a status symbol. Steak, prime rib, swordfish, sea bass and oysters are all celebratory, high end foods. Potatoes, corn, sweet potatoes, lentils and quinoa are still not considered upper class or high end!

Chapter 4: Working Out Doesn't Work

It is rather ironic that Americans are sick and fat and have simultaneously made the fitness industry a multibillion dollar industry. It just doesn't make sense! If fitness centers, equipment manufacturers, fitness "guru" DVDs and boot camp creators are so successful, why is the health of this country at an ALL TIME LOW?

Never before in history have we, as a society, ever been this unhealthy. Healthcare costs are soaring, life expectancy is decreasing and yet the fitness industry is booming. Think about that- the fitness industry is booming at a time when we are at an all time low in terms of our health!!

Have you walked into a fitness center lately? If not, just walk into L.A. Fitness and look around. Take note of how many overweight and obese people you see. At first, you may think" good for them, they are working on improving themselves."   Engage in a conversation with just a few of them and you will soon discover, they have been working out for years- many at that fitness center.

The cold hard fact is nothing has changed- he or she has been overweight for years! So what is going on? All of the marketing and the hype boldly state that working out, exercising like a lunatic will give you the sculpted, toned, trim body you always wanted. If this is the case, how is it some people will work out for 2-3 hours per day and still carry an extra 20, 30 even 40+ pounds? Some fitness experts would have you believe there is some miraculous combination of cardio and weights that leads to you arriving at your ideal weight.

Results speak for themselves, look around, do boot camps and gym memberships solve any weight issue? **There is a missing piece**. Exercise is not the cornerstone of optimal health. Then what is? *What is so undeniably crucial to health that without this cornerstone it is IMPOSSIBLE to achieve optimal health?* **The answer is the food you eat! That's right, it's all about your nutrition!**

There is no magic pill, wrap, energy drink, protein mix or post work out recovery drink that takes the place of the foundational nutrients you consume DAILY. Put junk in and your health is junk! Health revolves around the food that you eat. Exercise is absolutely a key lifestyle choice that supports the heart, lungs, joints, muscles and every other organ in the body. Exercise is very important- it is just not the reason you're overweight and sick... Below are the 7 fads the fitness industry doesn't want you to know....

1.) Exercise is the Calorie Bargaining Chip- Counting calories doesn't work. If it did, you would just simply be able to starve yourself for several days and lose weight. We know for a fact this never happens. It is not about calories. I guarantee someone who eats 2500 calories per day of fast food, macaroni and cheese, beer, hot dogs, cake and chicken wings – and does this on a daily basis- weighs significantly more than the person who eats 2500 calories per day of whole food, plant based foods such as fruits, vegetables, quinoa, rice, potatoes, sweet potatoes, nuts and seeds. **It is not the number of calories it is the quality of nutrients**.

So, going to the gym in the morning and running an extra 45 minutes on the treadmill to burn the extra calories so you can eat foolishly all day does not work! Results speak for themselves.

2.) Load up On the Protein To Build Lean Muscle and Lose Weight..... Animal protein- this includes fish, chicken, red meat, eggs and dairy- **is at the center of most disease processes.** It also, unfortunately is at the center of every nutrition conversation taking place at the gym. The absolute lie, fallacy, total untruth that many trainers, fitness gurus, gym rats and body builders spread as gospel is eat more protein so you can build more lean muscle.

You will look great, feel great and be as trim and toned as ever! There is absolutely no REAL, UNBIASED scientific evidence that supports building health through increased amounts of animal protein. One of the rarely spoken of dangers with high protein intake is the incredible disaster the amino acid, methionine, creates.

Methionine is found in high quantities in animal protein. The issue with this amino acid isf it destroys the epithelial layer of cells in blood vessels. The epithelial cells are responsible for producing nitric oxide which is the body's natural mechanism for lowering blood pressure. Ever wonder why so many big muscle guys and gals have high blood pressure when they work out 3-4 hours per day? It's simply too much methionine. High protein=high disease. **You will NEVER sustain health on a high protein diet.**

3.) Recipe For Disaster- Workouts must be fueled. Ask any professional athlete, before training or competition, pre game or pre training meals are as much a part of the workout as the exercise. Do you truly believe a professional football player shows up for practice hoping he has enough energy and stamina to make it through practice?

Of course not! It is far too common in many fitness centers to see people drinking energy drinks just as they are about to hop onto the treadmill. As a matter of fact, many fitness centers SELL energy drinks encouraging patrons to get "their energy for their workouts" from a can of poison! Energy does not come from artificially sweetened energy drinks.

Your energy for your workout comes from the food you eat. Want to fuel your workout? Have a banana, Clementine or strawberry and chia seed smoothie and you will have endless energy to run, bike or workout. Energy drinks are deadly. They are a lethal combination of stimulants! Want the recipe for a heart attack, at any age? Energy drink+ total dehydration (from not drinking water on a regular basis)+high acid/high protein/high inflammation in the body + strenuous exercise=the body's collapse- your kidneys and cardiovascular system do not have a chance!!!!

4.) Sports drinks are essential for replacing electrolytes and enhancing your workout! Totally false!!! Sports drinks have as much nutrition as a can of soda. That is correct! There is nothing nutritious or advantageous about most commercial sports drinks. First and foremost, they contain artificial sweeteners that are toxic to the body, especially the nervous system. Good, healthy, whole plant based food choices before and after your workout means the only drink you need while exercising is water! This holds true for those of you who exercise outdoors. Water, water and more water is what you need during strenuous exercise.

5.) Paleo + working out= fat and sick!.... There is not a greater stage for fad dieting than the fitness arena. Many fitness facilities call it the "total package"= high protein deadly food plus a gym membership. The proper food and nutrition is the cornerstone of health and the key to fighting disease.

Your food choices must be whole food, plant based, STARCH LOADED. **This no carb, low carb is completely false.** The research strongly supports only one way of healthy living and that is giving the body the nutrients it was meant to utilize which is starch first!! Dr. T. Colin Powell did a brilliant job delivering all of the research and proof anyone needs in his book, *The China Study*, proving time and time again through many research studies that animal protein promotes disease.

Eating steak, eggs, turkey, chicken, fish and dairy DOES NOT produce more lean muscle and it does not assist you in long term weight control. Muscle growth and development depends on the amino acids available in the body. These amino acids are strung together to make protein. We make some of those amino acids, others we must get from food. Well, **the most readily available amino acids in our diets come from plants**!! Plant based foods are very easy to digest, thus, making those precious amino acids readily available! The next huge

34

danger with animal products is the amount of saturated fat found in them. In fact, the saturated fat that is naturally found in all animal products is one of the main culprits in weight gain. You will wear your fat- it is that simple. The high amounts of fat are certainly the culprit in skyrocketing cholesterol and the risk for type II diabetes and cancer. Think about this, chicken breast is the breast tissue of another animal. Why would you think this is a low fat, lean protein?

6.) Increase the intensity, burn the fat....You can be super intense burning everything in sight and should you decide to consume a high fat diet, you will wear it! As so simply stated by Dr.John McDougall, "you wear your fat!"(9) .

The man belly, the spare tire, the double chin- it is all the result of poor nutrition. I do not know of anyone who eats a whole food, plant based, starch centered diet, exercises daily, sleeps 7-8 hours each night, stays hydrated and takes 2 tablespoons of apple cider vinegar and then one morning wakes up fat because the exercise intensity was too low!

High intensity interval training and high intensity exercise is certainly beneficial. However, it not nor will it ever be the excuse to eat and drink in total over indulgence and still maintain your optimal health and ideal weight.

7.) Fat burners accelerate weight loss- no MLM gimmicks, no infomercial gimmicks. There is no such thing as a fat burner in a bottle. You cannot eat junk, take a pill and sit on the couch watching the fat just melt right off your body! Regardless of the hype seen on TV and the crazy ads in the gyms or my personal favorite- all of the direct selling shakes plastered all over social media-there is no magic pill or shake! Think for just a moment.

It sounds too good to be true. Eat the worst food possible, add one shake per day or take a handful of junky supplements, then off to exercise and you look great, feel great and have perfect blood work. It is never going to happen! It is not about the exercise or the fat burner. It all hinges on the food you eat on a daily basis. Having trouble losing weight? Don't like the results of what you have been doing for the last decade? The answers are not increasing fat burners and spend an extra hour on the treadmill. The answer is let's fine tune your entire food plan!! Every single meal you eat has a result. It will have an effect on your liver, digestive system, heart, lungs, brain, kidneys, thyroid and skin. There is a result, the food you consume will determine if the result is a positive, health building result or a negative destructive, disease inviting result.

Let's recap! Exercise, working out is not a bargaining chip. Exercise is certainly a crucial part of a healthy lifestyle. However, it is not the cornerstone. By this I mean, your health does not revolve around exercise. The cornerstone of health- the bedrock which your health is supported is the nutrition from the food you eat. The fitness industry is an enormously profitable industry. Armed with biased fraudulent research, their deceptive advertising will have you believe that it's all about the exercise. It's not! Achieving optimal health and weight control is truly driven by what you eat. Remember, the only thing you are guaranteed to have with you until the day you leave planet earth is your health. It is time to build a lifestyle that promotes health. Eating a whole food plant based, starch loaded food plan is incredible. There are so many delicious foods- there is no deprivation at all!!

Chapter 5:   Is Your Environment Toxic?

Would you knowingly use a product everyday if you knew it would have very hazardous effects on your health? Would you do whatever it takes to protect your family from poison? The answers to these questions are quite obvious. However, our society seems to be blindly using products daily which are truly toxic.

Well, one of the most dangerous household toxins is ubiquitous- you cannot help but come in contact with it. This dangerous, health destroying, disease promoting threat is plastic. The safety of plastics is a hot topic in the research and health world. There are very valid concerns and negative health trends attributed to plastics. This is a topic that affects each and every one of us. So what is so terrible about plastic?

I am not suggesting that if you walk over to your food processor and touch the plastic on it you will spontaneously disintegrate. The problem is not with all plastic. The issue lies with the amount of plastic that comes in contact with our food and beverages. The one fatal flaw with many types of plastic is when plastic is heated; chemicals leach out of the plastic.

Heating breaks the plastic into many of its component parts. Some of those components are catastrophic to our health. The major concern is not have you ever come in contact with chemicals leached from plastic. All of us have and the body, just as it can do with other toxic substances, can neutralize these components with minimal damage. The real harm comes from the repeated daily exposure to harmful chemicals.

What plastics do you use daily? Plastics are common, found in most aspects of life. They are lightweight, easy to produce and relatively inexpensive. Most, if not all, common household items utilize plastic. The most obvious and frequently used products are water bottles, milk containers, yogurt cups, sandwich bags, condiment bottles, frozen food packaging, takeout food containers and coffee cups. Plastic has the massive potential to contaminate most of our foods.

The danger plastic presents lies in the ingredients used to produce plastic. Certain ingredients in plastics, notably the two most noxious offenders- bisphenol A (BPA) and 4-nonylphenol (NPH), are the most toxic to our food. These ingredients find their way in to our food once plastic is heated.

Hence, once you eat or drink from a plastic container or plastic water bottle that has been heated and the BPA or NPH has found its way into your food, you will consume the toxic substances. Why are these substances such a major health concern?

Well, these particular chemicals act as xenoestrogens. Xenestrogen are chemicals which act like the body's natural estrogen. However, they are far from friendly, they are foreign toxic chemicals. Xenoestrogens function like estrogen in that *they send hormonal signals to other cells in the body while simultaneously breaking down in to very poisonous waste which will harm the body*. By acting like estrogen, the plastics prevent your natural estrogen from functioning like it should.

Xenoestrogens have a terrible effect on the endocrine (hormonal) system. *Thyroid issues, fertility issues, breast issues, uterine issues, adrenal issues and other reproductive health issues are all heavily influenced by the toxic plastic byproducts.* It is commonly thought and supported by research that the increase in feminization (developing breast tissue) in our young males is directly related to the toxins in plastics.

Knowing xenoestrogens are so toxic, and that they trick our body into thinking they are estrogen begs the question, how much are plastics to blame for the increase in estrogen dominance issues in women? Breast cancer, hormonal imbalance, ovarian cysts and other issues related to the overabundance of estrogen may be directly related to the prolonged overexposure to xenoestrogens!

So, who is at the greatest risk? Quite simply, everyone!! Xenoestrogens are very harmful in both men and women. Perhaps, the most at risk population is our young-especially infants and children. Their systems are growing and developing so rapidly that the slightest disruption can have permanent devastating effects.

Most baby bottles and toddler cups contain BPA. As moms, it is crucial to look for cups, bottles, pacifiers, teething rings, utensils and toys which are BPA and NPH free. BPA and NPH are harmful to the nervous system. In a growing and developing child, the nervous system is delicate.

In addition to acting as xenoestrogens, BPA and NPH are also neurotoxins-substances toxic to the nervous system. That means even small repeated exposures can have a long term negative effect.

BPA and NPH are not just toxic to the nervous systems of the young. They also can wreck havoc in adults too. BPA and NPH have proven to be very irritating and harmful to the coverings of nerves. Degenerative disorders such as MS, rheumatoid arthritis, Lupus, Hashimotos and other brain, nervous system or autoimmune issues are certainly sensitive to these toxic chemicals.

Increasing the amounts of BPA and NPH in the system of someone with Lupus could certainly worsen the illness. Research also strongly suggests that eliminating these toxins from the lives of individuals with ADD, ADHD, autism, bipolar, depression, schizophrenia and other brain issues would be greatly beneficial in reducing symptoms.

This disturbing trend of estrogen issues in young men and women is senseless and can be stopped. Women with a high risk of breast cancer or those who have survived breast cancer should stop the use of all plastics which come in contact with food.

With concerns over the safety of some of the ingredients in plastic at an all time high, it is vital to know exactly what chemicals are found in the different types of plastics. Fortunately, all plastics are rated using a simple number system.

This categorization is for recycling purposes. This system is simple and uniform. It does not change from city to city or state to state. These numbers are found in a small triangle on the bottom of the container.

Understanding what plastics belong in each category and what danger each category poses is crucial information. This incredible health building knowledge allows you to avoid potentially toxic plastics. Using the system to your benefit is quite simple.

Remember, we are only concerned with plastic coming into contact with food. For example, let's use a container of peanut butter. Look on the bottom of the peanut butter and locate the number in the triangle. Check the information listed below to determine whether or not this particular container is safe for use with food. Below is all of the information you need on the categories of plastics.

Number One- Polyethylene Terephthalate (PET)- This plastic is common in many single use items such as salad dressings, mouthwashes, shampoos, hand sanitizers, stir fry sauces. Number one plastics are easy to recycle and are not known to leach chemicals into food. These items are not to be reused. Single use means once the container is empty it should be recycled. Should you see the number one in the triangle on your food item, you should feel comfortable using the product.

Number Two; High Density polyethylene (HDPE): This plastic is typically used for containers such as milk jugs, juice containers, tubs of butter and other food packaging. This is considered a very safe plastic and is easy to recycle. Number two plastics are considered stable and are not known to leach any chemicals into food. Again, as with ANY plastic, they are single use only! Do not keep the container and wash it and continue to reuse it. They will break down with repeated exposures to the heat of washing. One and done!

Number Three- Polvinyl Chloride or PVC- this particular category is used for plastics for cleaning agents, shower curtains, plastics for deli meats and many cling wraps. Number three plastics ARE NOT safe when used with food. They contain the chemical di2-ethylhexyl phthalate which is a known carcinogen! Also, these products contain chlorine or chlorine derivatives and should never come in contact with your food!

Number Four- Low Density Polyethylene (LDPE); this plastic is used in squeezable bottles, frozen food bags, grocery bags and storage bags. Number four is considered safe.

Number Five-Polypropylene (PP); This plastic is found in items such as medications, over the counter remedies, supplements (just a side note- all of the supplements in my office are dispensed in glass- no plastic used!!) straws, bottle caps, utensils and cups. This plastic is a sturdy plastic and meant for items that are not reused. You can feel safe using products with number 5, they are not known to leach chemicals into the contents of the packaging.

Number Six- Polystyrene (PS) This plastic is very hard and sturdy and is used for items that must maintain their form such as cups, toys, CD/DVD cases and take out containers. Polystyrene is also a component in foam and insulation. Number six plastics ARE NOT considered safe. They contain the chemical benzene which is very toxic and a known carcinogen. This means you MUST use extreme caution when eating out of take out containers- they can indeed leach chemicals into your food! Remember, the danger with plastic is when it is heated! How often are you picking up your take out food and it is steaming hot in the container .

Number Seven- "Other"; Yes, there is actually a category which contains plastics that contain a mixture of chemicals- most of them are harmful. Most plastics in number seven contain Bisphenol A which is highly toxic, a known xenoestrogen and wrecks havoc on the endocrine system. Category seven IS NOT safe, be very careful! This group includes plastics used in baby bottles, five gallon water or juice containers, sports drink bottles, microwave containers, liners for metal cans (Note; if a can of soup, vegetables, etc is organic, the liner of the can does not contain dangerous chemicals). Do not use number 7!!

Let's recap! What is the adequate margin of safety for the use of plastics? That has not been determined. To minimize, eliminate where possible, the use of plastics will only benefit your health! Here is what you can do to keep you and your family safe!

*Avoid ALL plastics with the codes 3,6,7**. They should never be in contact with your food or beverages. No questions asked, just move on and find another product.

*Use 1,2,4 and 5 with caution**. Never reuse or apply any type of heat to plastic and then consume the contents! This applies to microwave too.

*Use alternatives such as glass or stainless steel water bottles, glass dishes and storage containers**. Always use glass in the microwave! Many juices come in glass containers. Save the container, wash it out and you have another water bottle.

*STOP BUYING BOTTLED WATER- if the majority of water you drink is bottled water, you are creating a massive health problem!!   NEVER drink a bottle of water and then refill it and keep using it!

*Educate yourself on the system. Some companies will use the abbreviations of the plastic and not a number in the triangle. For example, PP may appear on a container instead of the number 5.

* This is an area where **consistency adds up**- for good or bad!

    Just to make sure you are clear, plastic is a danger when it is heated and dangerous chemicals leach into your food or beverage. Realize that many products sit on delivery trucks and in warehouses that reach stifling temperatures. Some bottled water, sports drinks and other foods and drinks in plastic can reach temperatures of 150-160 degrees locked in a delivery truck or storage facility. This is enough heat to cause a breakdown of the plastic components and cause the contamination and danger.

    Take this seriously; this is precisely why bottled water and sports drinks are so unhealthy. Do you routinely bring a bottle of water in the car and leave it there why you do your shopping, go to work, etc?

    Living in a world of convenience can be incredibly dangerous for your health. Take this information and spend some time evaluating the safety of your food and beverages. Make simple changes!!

Chapter 6:   Just In- Study Confirms This Sweetener *Unleashes* Toxins...

Sucralose is another name springing up on plenty of food labels. It sounds fine- you may have even confused it with fructose or sucrose. Well, sucralose is the evil cousin of high fructose corn syrup and aspartame. Sucralose is more commonly known as **_Splenda!_** Yes indeed, it is another deadly artificial sweetener.

Many food producers in response to the outrage (and rightfully so!) of aspartame, have replaced it with sucralose. Sucralose is very sweet and of course is deemed safe by the FDA in small amounts. It is found in foods such as sports drinks, flavored water, iced teas, soda, fruit juices and drinks, cookies, cakes, granola bars, cereals, breads, ice cream, trail mix, candy and gum*. It is even added to children's medicines, vitamins and over the counter cold remedies.*

So, what risk does sucralose pose? Make no mistake, sucralose is a chemical sweetener. It does not exist anywhere in nature- it is totally manufactured! It contains harsh chemicals, the worst of which is chlorine. That is right, chlorine!

Now chlorine is very reactive and by the way, a favorite of food chemists. Many scientists have insisted sucralose does not cross the blood brain barrier like aspartame does, therefore it does not damage the nervous system. So, how could it be harmful?

Unfortunately, sucralose does contain carcinogenic chemicals and the body is exposed to these chemicals.

Once you ingest a toxin, you expose plenty of the gastrointestinal system and other of the body's systems to harsh toxic chemicals. The body must breakdown and neutralize anything toxic,. Research shows that 10-15 % of sucralose remains in the digestive tract and may possibly be stored in the body!!

Think about that for a second, every time your child drinks a sports drink, eats potato chips or a candy bar, the most toxic by product may stay in his growing maturing body!!

In Depth Scientific Review....Lies Exposed

For years Splenda has been the best selling artificial sweetener in the world. That's right, in the world. It is touted to be safe and effective for diabetics and those who are obese and searching for weight reduction.

Research now supports what has long been suspected by natural doctors for years, Splenda worsens booth diabetes and obesity. Furthermore, Splenda is associated with plenty of other health issues. An in depth scientific review of Splenda published in the *Journal of Toxicology and Environmental Health* reveals an entire laundry list of potentially devastating safety concern for Splenda.

The safety concerns include toxicity, DNA damage, demolition of health gut flora and increase in carcinogenic potential when heated- these are just a few!!! The destruction of the gut flora is catastrophic to your health. When the gut doesn't function well, the rest of the body will start to break down. This alone should be enough for families to STOP BUYING foods that contain sucralose.

Be on the look out for sucralose!

Sucralose is an artificial sweetener. It is used to replace sugar in many foods. Its **sole purpose is to sweeten or add flavor.** Sucralose is cheap and easy to make. It is a favorite of many food manufacturers.

You will find sucralose in candy bars, sports drinks, granola bars, cookies, cakes, juices, brownies, ice cream, breads, soda, dried fruits, canned fruits, children's vitamins, children's medicines and flavored water. This is only a small list of the most common offenders. Develop the habit of reading your food label.

See what is used to sweeten the food.(Even better-start eating one ingredient foods and prepare your food at home- stop buying processed food!) What are the first three or four ingredients? These ingredients make up at least 80% of the food. Ingredients are listed in descending order of % content. Meaning, the first ingredient listed is in the highest concentration in that product.

For example, if the first ingredient listed is whole wheat flour, it is a predominately made up of whole wheat flour. In many cases, artificial sweeteners will be the third or fourth ingredient. Become an ingredient detective- always read the nutrition label!

Of course, eating fresh fruits and vegetables is best. Mother nature produces many sweet treats! *"If God did not make it then don't eat it"* is one of Jack LaLanne's famous quotes and words he truly lived by!

Many natural or organic food manufacturers use natural sweeteners such as brown rice syrup, fruit puree, agave, coconut water and honey. You can be healthy and enjoy great taste. Here is one final hint, the fewer ingredients on a label, the better the product!

What's the harm?

Sucralose or "Splenda" as it is better known, is a chemical substance- it is a foreign substance in the body. The problem with sucralose is roughly 15% of it ingested will be absorbed into the body. This means it will have an opportunity to expose other healthy tissue to a toxic substance.

If you were to break down sucralose, one of the byproducts would be chlorine. Many health professionals have very serious concerns about the chlorine and for good reason. The FDA deems chlorine so harmful they have been pushing the paper industry to remove chlorine from the paper making process! So far, it has not worked.

Think about what chlorine does, it gets whites whiter! Do you want that substance left in your body? Remember, what is absorbed more than likely will be stored. Chlorine is not a chemical that should be left to roam the body! Studies have shown sucralose will worsen the symptoms of Lupus, MS, rheumatoid arthritis, worsening of food allergies, Crohn's disease and Fibromyalgia.

The most devastating result of artificial sweeteners, including sucralose, is it will destroy close to fifty percent (50%) of your gut's natural flora from repeated exposures. That's right, keep consuming artificial sweeteners and one of the biggest defense systems your body has will be annihilated! A growing concern with sucralose use, as well as other artificial sweeteners and food dyes, is the amount of them added to foods that our young kids eat. The diets of children contain artificial sweeteners starting from birth!!

Those infants who use infant formula may be exposed to sucralose, aspartame or some other artificial sweeteners! Can you imagine by the time a child reaches 18, his body will have metabolized some of the most dangerous chemicals and some of the most dangerous carcinogens! Repeated exposure to dangerous chemicals for nearly eighteen years- no wonder our kids are suffering from adult health issues such as high blood pressure and type II diabetes at remarkably young ages! **Remember, there is a nutritional component to every disease!**

Oh, my aching muscles!

Sports drinks, muscle builders, protein drinks and sports recovery drinks are everywhere! Their popularity is only second to bottled water. The biggest problem is the more popular brands are nothing more than chemistry experiments! They are filled with artificial sweeteners and dyes.

Sucralose is a very popular sweetener used in protein mixes, mass building supplements, muscle recovery drinks and electrolyte replacement drinks. Many athletes, believing they are doing what is right, consume these drinks before during and after athletic performances. The sucralose will cause muscle cramping, aches and pains.

Remember, your body recognizes sucralose as an intruder. It will work harder to get rid of sucralose **before** it will use those mighty amino acids to build muscle! Also, the detox required will likely deplete some of your vital water stores, leading to a post workout dehydration.

So, if you are suffering from muscle soreness, increased muscle fatigue or muscle cramping while engaging in strenuous exercise, check the label of your muscle/protein drink- I bet it contains sucralose! Water still remains the best hydrator! Look for products not sweetened with sucralose, or any other artificial sweetener- cannot find any, then make your own!!! It is quite simple- water with fresh lemon, lime and a pinch of salt and stevia!

Chapter 7: How would you like to live off pizza, pasta, tacos and burritos?

We have spent the last several chapters discussing foods that lead to disease. Now, let's move on to some fun stuff! Eating healthy which arms the body with the vitamins and nutrients needed to destroy disease is actually incredibly delicious. No starvation, no deprivation on this meal plan! There is so much food available to eat daily, you will never feel like you are "on a diet". In this chapter, you will find a pantry make over list as well as some of my favorite quick and easy to make recipes. So, let's eat!

The first step in your health transformation is preparation. The following items are the staples-the basic fundamentals- for every plant powered health building pantry.

Perishables:

Potatoes	Lemons	Rice or almond milk
Spinach	Soy/ tamari sauce	
Garlic	Sweet Potatoes	Almonds/ cashews
Basil	Veggie Burger (no soy protein isolate)	
Onions	Avocado	Chia seeds
Parsley	Corn/Rice Wrap	
Bananas	Tomatoes	Berries
Salsa	Jam	
Hummus	Sprouted bread/bagels	Pizza crust/dough
Pitas	Maca powder	

Non-Perishables:

Brown Rice
Quinoa

Organic Canned Black Beans
Nutritional Yeast

Rice pasta
Ketchup/Mustard

Organic Canned Chick Peas

Organic canned tomatoes
Flour (unbleached)

Dry kidney and black beans

Organic marinara sauce
Honey

Vegetable Broth

Green/Herbal Tea
Peanut butter

Organic coffee/ganoderma

Hot sauce
Popcorn

Oats/oatmeal

Herbs and Spices

Sea salt
Nutmeg

Onion powder
Oregano

Pepper
Chili Powder

garlic powder
cinnamon

Bay leaves
Turmeric

Vanilla Extract
Vegetable Seasoning mix

Basil

Crushed Red Pepper

Paprika

**Bonus – A must need for your kitchen is a high powered blender such as the nutri-bullet . This versatile blender will be the workhorse of your menu. Responsible for your delicious health building smoothies, a nutri- bullet also can be used as a mini food processor, assisting with making soups, flours, pancakes and desserts.

Get Ready, Get Set, Get Eating...

Now that you have gotten rid of all of the dairy, chicken, fish and red meat, here are your yummy plant powered replacements. Before we jump into the menus, I want to give you 7 basic success strategies that will assist you in making this awesome transformation.

1.) The first rule is, there are no rules!! You can have rice and beans for breakfast and pancakes for dinner! Break the restricting mindset of breakfast foods, lunch foods and dinner foods. Food is fuel and nourishment and it cannot tell time! The focus will be on the quality of nutrition.

2.) You must drink plenty of water each and every day. Hydration is crucial. Your water intake must be 3-4 quarts per day.

3.) Enjoy all of the fruit and vegetables you want.

4.) Avoid using excess fats such as oils, margarines, butters- even vegetable oils and olive oils.

5.) Use minimally processed soy foods. For example, soy burgers, cheeses, tofu should not be part of your daily food plan, they should be used sparingly.

6.) Choose the least processed starches available. For example, sprouted bread is a better choice than commercial wheat bread. Always use fresh starches whenever possible. French fries are not the same nutritionally as a baked potato.

7.) Include starch with every meal. Fresh plant based starches such as potatoes, squash, rice, sweet potatoes and quinoa are incredible and are the cornerstone of your transformation.

Bonus Start each and every day with 2 tablespoons of apple cider vinegar in a few ounces of water.

Dr.Christa's 18 Favorite, Simple, Plant Powered Recipes

I hate to cook; however, I do know how to make delicious, healthy foods that the entire family will love. All of my recipes are simple, quick to prep and cook and loaded with flavor and nutrition....enjoy!

Smoothies

Smoothies are a great way to get a bunch of fruits and veggies in. For those of you who are not a huge fan of greens such as spinach, kale and beet greens; smoothies are the perfect hiding place for your daily serving of greens! They are quick, easy to make and very portable. I suggest using smoothies as part of a meal and also as a delicious snack.

Anti-Inflammatory-eases pain, boosts the heart and is great after a workout

1 cup of spinach
1 cup of pineapple
1 cup of berries
1/3 of a fresh beet, peeled- chop the stems and add them too.
2 teaspoons of chia seeds
1 teaspoon of maca powder

Put all ingredients in nutri bullet or blender, fill with water and enjoy!

Stomach Soother:

1 cup of fresh pineapple
½ cup of papaya
1 kiwi- peeled

Put all ingredients in a nutri bullet or blender, fill with water and enjoy.

Super Green Detoxer:
1 cup of spinach-
2 stalks of celery
½ cucumber
¼ of a lemon- with the rind on
1 tsp. of chia
(for extra detox add 1 tsp. of spiralina)

Put all ingredients in a nutri-bullet or blender, fill with water and enjoy.

Mega anti oxidant cooler

1 cup of pineapple
1 cup of strawberries
1 teaspoon of chia seeds
1 tsp. of maca powder

Put all ingredients in a nutria- bullet or blender, fill with water and enjoy.

Peanut Butter & Chocolate Dream

*This is one of my favorite post run drinks!
It is filling and great after a long work out or
on your way to work!!!

1 cup of fresh spinach
4-5 dates (pitted)
5 strawberries
1 banana
1-2 tblsp. of peanut butter
1 tsp. of cacoa or carob powder
1 cup of rice milk

Put all ingredients in a nutria-bullet or blender, add extra
water if necessary, blend and enjoy.

Plant Based Main Dishes

Pasta, Bean & Tomato Stew

(1) 28 oz. can of organic tomatoes
(1) -12-14oz package of elbow or ditalini
1/2 red pepper- chopped
1/2 onion- chopped
3-4 cloves of garlic
1 can of organic chick peas - rinsed
4 bay leaves
6-8 fresh basil leaves
1-2 tsp. Italian seasoning
3cups of water

Place onion, garlic, red pepper.chick peas,
uncooked macaroni, Italian seasoning,
basil leaves, bay leaves, water and tomatoes
 in a pot or skillet. Fill empty

tomato can with water and add water
to the pot. Cook on high until liquid
starts to boil. Turn down heat and
let simmer on low to medium heat.
Stir frequently. Mixture will thicken
as pasta cooks. Allow to cook
for 10-20 minutes, serve with a
side salad or a side of asparagus
or broccoli and enjoy!!!

Potato and tomato stew

6-8 golden potatoes peeled and cut into chunks
1 can of Muir tomatoes (I use the fire roasted with garlic)
1 cup of organic frozen peas
1 cup of organic frozen corn
1/2 white onion- chopped
2 cloves of fresh garlic (mince with garlic press)
2 tablespoons of nutritional yeast
salt and pepper
1/2 tablespoon of olive oil

Place potatoes in a pot of water, cover and let come to a
boil. Let potatoes boil for 5-7 minutes until tender. Drain
water from pot. Sprinkle the nutritional yeast on potatoes,
mix and set the pot aside. In a large skillet, heat olive oil.
Add chopped onion and fresh garlic. Let onions and garlic
heat until tender and slightly brown. Add tomatoes,
reduce heat, cover and let cook on low- medium heat for
5-7 minutes. Add peas and corn, mix well. Add cooked
potatoes, mix well. Add salt and pepper to taste. Let the
skillet heat on low for 10-15 minutes.

This dish is quick, easy and delicious!! It is also very
versatile- you can use whatever veggies you have in the

refrigerator. I also love to add spinach to this dish- go ahead and try it!!!

Banana Pancakes

1 ¼ cup of oat
½ cup of organic whole wheat or oat flour
½ tsp. sea salt
2 ripe bananas
1 1/2 cups of soy or rice milk

Mash bananas in a medium bowl and set aside.
Mix oats, flour, salt in a large bowl. Slowly add
soy milk to flour mixture. Mix contents so mixture
is batter like. Add bananas to the batter and mix. Heat
griddle or frying pan, spray with a small amount of
non-stick cooking spray. Place a small amount of batter
on the griddle. Let the pancake cook until the edges are
firm,
flip and allow to cook through. Serve immediately with
fresh
maple syrup.

Butternut Squash and Pasta Soup

1 butternut squash, peel and cube
1 onion- chopped
2 tomatoes- diced
1 can of tomato sauce- (small can)
1 1/2 cups of dry fettuccine or spaghetti, broken into 2-3
inch pieces -organic pasta!
Salt and pepper to taste
1 cup of veggie broth or dry cooking wine

Cook onion in the wine or broth until tender. Put in a
blender and blend until smooth. Return mixture to the pot

and heat. Add the tomato and tomato sauce. Let the mixture simmer for about 10 minutes. Add the squash, cook for another 5-7 minutes. Add pasta to the mixture and cook until the pasta is soft. Add additional broth or water if needed. Add salt and pepper and enjoy!!

No oil, no artificial sweeteners or dyes- just whole food plant based out of the world food!!!!!!

Cucumber, Avocado, Tomato Salad

1 cucumber, peeled and chopped
1 large tomato- chopped
1/2 red onion, sliced thin
1 avocado- remove skin and chop
1 lemon
Salt and Pepper

Gently mix the cucumber, tomato, onion
and avocado in a large bowl. Squeeze
the juice from the fresh lemon- it
will be about 2 tblsp. Add lemon juice
to bowl. Top with salt and pepper and enjoy!!

Black bean and corn salad

2 cans of black beans, drained and rinsed WELL
1 can fire roasted, diced tomatoes
1 package of frozen corn (16 oz.), thawed by running under warm water in drainer
1/2 purple onion, diced
1 can of water chestnuts, drained and rinsed
bunch cilantro, chopped
juice and zest from 1/2 lime
3+ Tbsps. balsamic vinegar, to suite your taste

Salt and garlic powder, to your taste
Mix lime juice, vinegar, salt and garlic powder together in small bowl. Combine remaining ingredients in large bowl. Mix in vinegar mixture, chill and enjoy!

Black Bean Burgers

1 can (15-16oz) of black beans
1/2 cup of fresh cilantro
1 onion
3-4 cloves of garlic
½ cup of cooked brown rice
Dash of cumin
Dash of hot sauce
1 ½ cup of bread crumbs

In food processor: Combine beans, cilantro, onion, garlic, egg and Worcestershire/hot sauce. Process until well blended and then pour into a bowl. Add bread crumbs, cumin and mix . Shape into patties. Bake 20 minutes at 375 degrees. ** The patties freeze well and make a great meal on those busy evenings or also make a great snack for the kids after school!!

Spinach and Bean Soup

1 32 oz. carton of vegetable broth
1 bag of fresh spinach
3 cloves of garlic, crushed
1 medium onion, chopped
2 cans of cannellini beans, unrinsed
3 tablespoons of olive oil
 In a large pan, heat oil. Sautee garlic and onion. Add beans and cook for 2-3 minutes. Add chicken broth and bring to a boil. Add spinach and cook until spinach has reduced and is tender. Serves 4. Add a side salad to make a low cal, fiber rich meal! This soup is even better the next day!!!!!

Mango Slaw With Cashews

2 Mangoes, peeled, pitted and chopped
1 to 1 ½ pounds of Napa cabbage sliced thin
1 red pepper chopped
½ red onion, chopped thin
6 tablespoons of fresh lime juice (the juice from 2 limes)
¼ cup rice vinegar
2 tablespoons of olive oil
Pinch of salt
¼ cup of cashews chopped
¼ tsp of red pepper flakes (omit if you do not like the heat!)

Toss mangoes, cabbage, red pepper and onion in large bowl. Whisk lime juice, oil, vinegar, salt and red pepper in smaller bowl. Pour dressing mixture over slaw. Sprinkle cashews on slaw- you can serve immediately or let it set in the refrigerator for an hour. Enjoy!!

Tomato and Bean Wrap:

2 cups of chopped tomatoes
1 can of organic black beans drained and rinsed
1 cup chopped avocado
½ cup of chopped red onion
2 tablespoons of lime juice
2 tablespoons of fresh chopped cilantro
Pinch of salt
Corn, or whole wheat tortillas or flatbread

Combine tomatoes, beans, avocado, onion, cilantro, lime juice in a bowl. Add a pinch of salt. Cover and refrigerate for ½ hour. Add a portion of the mixture to the tortilla, add lettuce if you like- enjoy!

Yummy Desserts:

Banana Ice Cream:

Slice 2-3 bananas and freeze
½ cup almond milk
Place frozen bananas in your nutri bullet
Add ¼-1/2 cup of almond milk
Blend, serve in a small bowl!
(Hint: Add your favorite berries!)

Peanut Butter Cookies
(Teenager tested, Dr.Christa approved)

1 ¼ cup chick peas
¾ cup of peanut butter
½ cup of honey
¼ teaspoon of baking soda
2 teaspoons of vanilla extract
½ cup of chocolate chips

Preheat oven to 350. Combine all ingredients, except the chocolate chips in a food processor. Mix until ingredients are well combined and the chick peas are blended smooth. Fold in the chocolate chips. Roll the cookie dough into balls and place on a non stick cookie sheet. Bake for 15-18 minutes, until bottom of cookies are brown. Enjoy!!

The first step in any healing and health transformation is optimizing your food plan. Vitamins, minerals and nutrients heal. The most powerful pharmacy in the world is the produce section of your local grocery store. That is the starting point. There is not a disease in existence that will not respond to an improvement in nutrition. Food is medicine- it was the first medicine ever used. Time will always tell its tale, food continues to be the most powerful weapon in fighting disease and building health.

Banana & Blueberry Bread

   3 ripe bananas
¼ cup of organic agave
3/4 tsp. of baking powder
3/4 tsp of baking soda
1/3 cup of soy or rice milk
2 tblsp. of juice of fresh lemon
1 cup of blueberries
1 cup of almond flour

Mix the nut milk and 1 tblsp. lemon juice together and set aside. Let it stand until it starts to sour or curdle. Mash bananas and 1 tblsp of lemon juice. Add soymilk and agave and blueberries. In a separate bowl mix the almond flour, baking soda and baking powder. Add the dry mixture slowly to the banana mixture. Mix until ingredients are well combined and it is on the "doughy" side. If necessary, add more almond flour. The mixture should not be too moist or your bread will be soggy. Once mixture is combined. Add the mixture to a bread pan. Bake at 350* for 50-60 minutes.

Chapter 8: This is the potential of implementing what I recommend—

Nine years ago, a wonderful and amazing woman was diagnosed with breast cancer. After the initial shock of the diagnosis, she followed the instructions given by her doctor. They of course included the "traditional" course of treatment of multiple lumpectomies, chemotherapy and a course of radiation. This was the "best" option available, or so she was told.

She was fully compliant enduring endless hours of pain, fatigue, nausea, vomiting, hair loss, skin changes and of course an immune system that was overtaken and opportunistic infections hit her one after another. She fought day in and day out. She completed her treatment and began to put her life back together.

She went for her follow up mammograms, blood work and ultrasounds to "make sure no new cancer was discovered." This went on for five years! Not once during this process did any doctor or nurse ever say to her, "let's take a look at your lifestyle and see where we can improve".

No one ever discussed food, exercise, sleep, stress reduction- all of the factors that make sure cancer cannot survive in the body. She was so close to that coveted 5 year cancer survivor marker- so close...... Then, it happened, another lump was found, in the same breast and it was once again, malignant breast cancer!

Convinced she could not survive the surgery and chemo again AND certainly convinced she had more living to do, she decided to explore alternative opportunities *to build her body and enable her body to fight the cancer*.

She assembled a a team of health professionals including me, primary care physician and an oncologist to monitor her blood work, MRI and ultrasound and several other team members- she was ready to change. She believed in the power of food and the body and the capabilities of the body when it is given the right nutrition.

Fast forward 4 years and her most recent scans show NO EVIDENCE OF HER PRIMARY TUMOR. *Her oncologist could not believe* it! This is an absolutely incredible health transformation. This woman is dedicated to herself and her health. ***If giving up the meat and dairy-switching to a whole food plant based diet can destroy breast cancer, what can it do for you?***

Fertility- No Issue

Many women dream of raising a family. It seems natural, "the way it's supposed to be". Well, for this particular patient, it was not going to be that easy. Previous ovarian cysts and an ectopic pregnancy, left this awesome young woman without the ability to get pregnant. Her only alternative was in vitro is not guaranteed.

This lengthy process involving medications and numerous medical procedures very often does not leave patients with the desired end result-pregnancy- after just 'one round". It could take many rounds, several years and tens of thousands of dollars. So, she said to me, what can we do to really get me ready for this and totally skyrocket my chances of a successful IVF the first time?

I immediately, put together what foods are best at nourishing the reproductive system, what foods need to be immediately eliminated because they disrupt the hormonal balance, a plan of attack using acupuncture and exercise recommendations. ***Fast forward 5 months and this incredible young lady is pregnant, her first IVF was a success!!!***

Total Chaos To Total Focus- Food Fights ADHD

After 65 years this woman had enough. Her health was miserable. At nearly 100 pounds overweight, taking 6-7 prescriptions per day, mood swings and irritability that affected every relationship in her life, unable to turn her racing thoughts off long enough to work effectively or sleep soundly; this patient knew life could not continue in such utter chaos.

Her food plan consisted of a steady diet of breakfast sausage, eggs, lunch meat, hamburgers, cheeseburgers and every drive-thru within a 10 mile radius. She spent decades consuming processed animal protein and high fat processed foods. It certainly did show! *There was no hiding obesity, lack of focus, mood swings and poor health.*

With so much going on where do we even start? That was the question she asked over and over. She tried many fad diet plans. So, we decided the starting point would be simple, drink water every day, take 2 tablespoons of apple cider vinegar and add 3-4 servings of fruits and vegetables daily. That was it that was the starting point.

Over the course of the next 15-18 months, this wonderful lady made small systematic changes to her food plan. She now has eliminated all meat, dairy, fish and chicken. She is purely plant powered, enjoying a wide range of fruits, veggies, grains and seeds.

Her health has dramatically changed. She is reducing her medication and will soon be medication free, she has more energy than ever before, her immune system is great, she no longer gets a sinus infection every other week.

Most impressively, she reports she can control her mood and focus like never before. She has never experienced the clarity and the calmness that she now has. She got rid of all of the junk! The brain is obviously a crucial part of our existence! You better believe that it needs the right fuel and nutrients to function.

In her own words, cardiologist shocked

Dr.Christa is definitely a nutrition expert. She helped me and my husband create a food plan to save our hearts and improve our health and I am certainly not disappointed.

As a matter of fact, I could not be happier. I know to bring my food and nutrition questions to Dr.Chirsta and let my cardiologist handle the medication. *My cardiologist has been amazed, almost in disbelief with the strides I have made by adding the right foods and getting rid of all of the dairy and fish.*

My cardiologist had me add fish and dairy and get rid of red meat a year ago and my blood work just kept getting worse and worse. I had a consult with Dr.Christa and the first thing she did was get rid of the dairy, fish and increase the sweet potatoes, beets, walnuts, spinach and other healthy foods. *It went totally against the initial advice my doctor gave me.*

Within four months my blood work had radically changed and I had more energy and less pains in my legs. That got me really excited! I meet with Dr.Christa every few weeks and we make the changes that need to be made. My blood work and health just keep getting better. Thank you Dr. Christa for being my food guide! You are the best!

These three patients have very different stories. The health challenges they face seem like they could not possibly have any common connection. Yet, it is proven time and again, the foundation to fight disease and achieve optimal health is the food you consume. These are extreme examples- extreme health transformations. ***Take a long look at what using food as medicine can do, imagine what it can do for you...***

For Nearly 20 Years, Dr.Christa has been changing lives, here's what others are saying......

"Thanks to you I can walk again! My hip and leg were in so much pain, I could barely get through the day. With your acupuncture and help, I feel great. Even my co-workers noticed! You care about me as a person.

No doctor has ever asked me if I want to get healthy enough to stop taking my blood pressure and cholesterol medication. I didn't even know that was possible! I am so excited I found you. For the first time in decades, I feel like I have a healthy future, I can't thank you enough!" *MD, Ft. Lauderdale, Fl.*

"I cannot believe it, the migraines are gone! Acupuncture is my miracle cure. I have been suffering from migraines that would leave me completely helpless, it almost cost me my job. I tried medication after medication after medication and the only thing that happened is I got so sick from the meds and still had to deal with the headaches.

After just 4 weeks, my headaches were under control. After 5 months they are just about gone. Thank you for cleaning up my food, I always thought I ate healthy and I guess I really didn't. You showed me how to improve my food and eat the right foods to make me feel great. Thank you for putting up with me and especially for giving me my life back!" *OLS, Coral Springs, FL*

But Wait...There's More...Here's A Special Bonus Article

What kills cancer cells, grows on trees and is in your refrigerator?

"My health has never been so great! Dr.Christa straightened out my food and put me on the right herbs. Now I feel like I did when I was 30!" L.L., Deerfield Beach

I have often said, there is a nutritional root to every disease. This is absolutely true. Foods have tremendous power- both good and bad. Many drug companies have recognized foods possess therapeutic power. The basis of many prescription drugs is indeed many plant and food components.

For example, statin drugs are replications of lovstatin, which is a component of red rice yeast and certain fungi. The effects of lovastatin in its natural form where noted in the early 1970's. The drug companies then took what nature produces and attempted to replicate it in a lab.

Then, voila, we have *Lipitor* and all of the other statin drugs!! What's wrong with red rice yeast and mushrooms??? Very simply, they are not very profitable! So, back to the title question... What grows on trees, is in your fridge and kills cancer cells? The answer is ***lemons!***

As I instruct each and every patient, water with lemon juice is a daily must do! Research, completed by the drug companies back in the 1970's, reveals that the juice of lemons has the ability to kill malignant cancer cells. (this research continues today!)

It is considered to be more powerful than drugs such as Adriamycin, and other chemotherapeutic agents. Studies show the juice of the lemon was effective in annihilating tumors of the breast, colon, ovaries and uterus. This is just incredible information!

One tablespoon of lemon juice in a glass of water taken several times per day- EVERYDAY- is a huge ally in the fight against cancer! The juice of the lemon is also an excellent anti microbial agent, killing many viruses, parasites, bacteria and fungi. So, what is in lemons that make them so powerful?

Well, everything! Lemons have many different antioxidants, are loaded with vitamins, minerals, flavinoids and other integral health compounds. It is impossible to isolate just one or two compounds that pack the power punch. Nature does not make junk- in its natural form, lemons are life saving!

How can you harness the power of lemons? Very simply, add fresh organic (no artificial coloring or sweeteners) lemons or lemon juice to your water everyday!! What day? EVERYDAY!!!

Make it easy on yourself, take one gallon of water, add ¼ cup of lemon juice to it and drink it daily! If you or someone you know is at risk for colon, breast, uterine or ovarian cancer – start drinking lemon juice everyday!

We are blessed here in south Florida, there is no shortage of lemons! Squeeze the juice of a fresh lemon in your water and enjoy!! Mother nature is simply incredible! Lemons are also a best friend for the liver. They have a very unique cleansing ability. Those of you with allergies, taking any type of medication, suffering from gall bladder issues or after an evening of too much alcohol, reach for lemons! Your liver will certainly thank you.

Of course, there is one more bonus when you drink water with lemon juice daily- you will reduce your risk of osteoporosis by more than 60%! That's right, lemon juice once digested, results in an alkaline ash. This keeps calcium, which is the body's first choice of buffers when things get too acidic, in the blood, bones and muscles where it belongs! You really cannot go wrong with lemons!!!!

One of my favorite ways to liven up any smoothie is to take a slice of lemon, with the rind on, and blend it in your smoothie!

References

(1)   Barzel US. "Excess dietary protein can adversely affect bone". Journal of Clinical Nutrition. 1998 June; 128(6): 1051-53

(2)   www.dairycheckoff.com

(3)   Yu,H and Rohan T. "Role of the Insulin like growth factor family in cancer development and progression" Journal of National Cancer Institute; 2000, Sept. 20; 92(18) p. 1472-89.

(4)   Morin RJ, Hu B, Peng SK, Sevanian A, Cholesterol Oxides and Carcinogens. Jour. Clini. Lab Anal. 1991; 5)3);219-25

(5)((Ahn J., AlbanesD, Peters U, et al. Prostate, Lung, Colorecal and Ovarian Trial Project Team. Dairy Products, calcium intake and risk of prostate cancer in the prostate, lung colorectal and ovarian cancer screening tiral *Cancer Epidemiol Biomarkers Prev.* 2007 Dec; 16 (12):2623-30.))

(6))Bruce ALberts, Alexander Johnson, Julian Lewis, Martin Raff, Keith Roberts, and Peter Walter. " Protein Function" *Molecular Biology of the Cell 4th Edition*

/) David Zieve, MD, MHA, and Dvid R Eltz. "Protein n diet" US National Library of Medicine, Department of Health and Human Services, National Institutes of Health.

(8)T.Collin Campbell, PhD. Thomas M. Campbell II, MD. *The China Study* .Benbella Books, 2006. P.28

(9) Dr.John McDougall, *The Starch Solution,* Rodale Inc., 2012. P.25.